Cow-Faced-Pose

Gomukhāsana

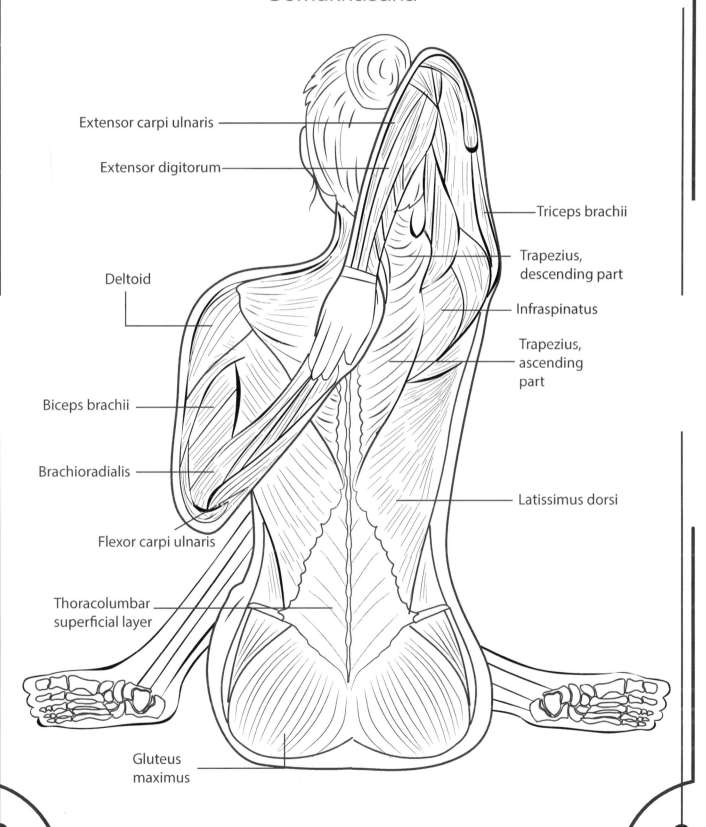

Extensor carpi ulnaris

Extensor digitorum

Triceps brachii

Trapezius, descending part

Deltoid

Infraspinatus

Trapezius, ascending part

Biceps brachii

Brachioradialis

Latissimus dorsi

Flexor carpi ulnaris

Thoracolumbar superficial layer

Gluteus maximus

Pigeon Pose

Eka-Pāda Rājakapotāsana

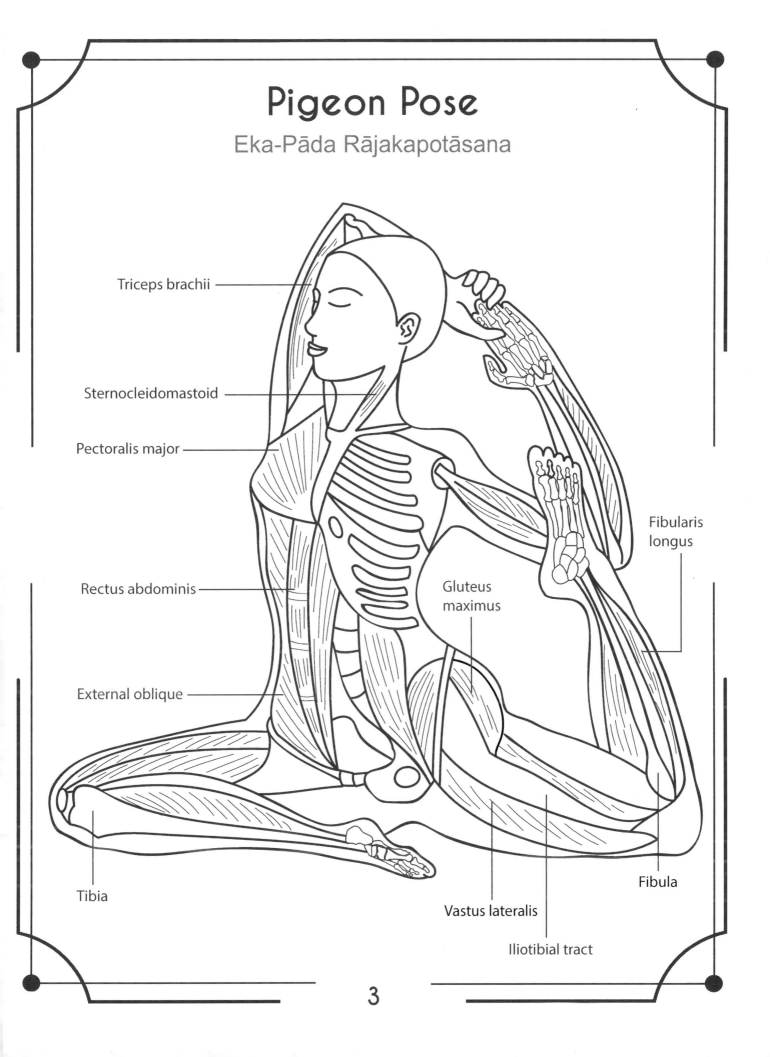

Triceps brachii

Sternocleidomastoid

Pectoralis major

Rectus abdominis

External oblique

Tibia

Gluteus maximus

Fibularis longus

Fibula

Vastus lateralis

Iliotibial tract

Triangle Pose

Trikoṇāsana

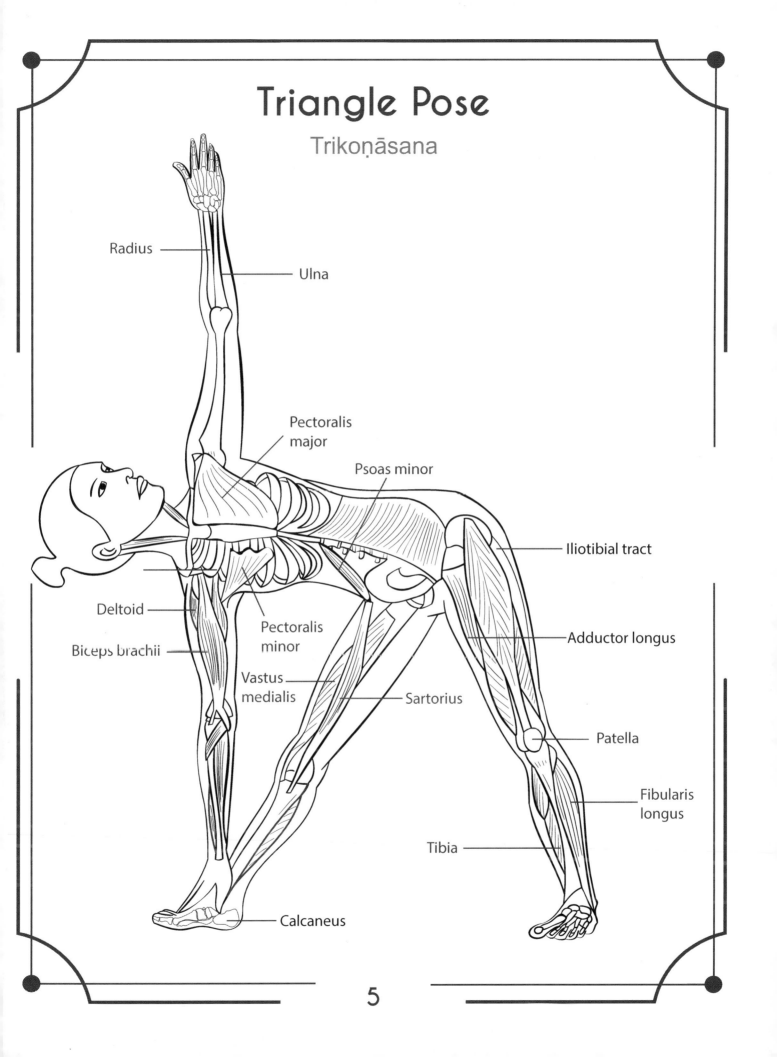

Radius

Ulna

Pectoralis
major

Psoas minor

Iliotibial tract

Deltoid

Pectoralis
minor

Biceps brachii

Adductor longus

Vastus
medialis

Sartorius

Patella

Fibularis
longus

Tibia

Calcaneus

Bound Angle Pose

Baddha Koṇāsana

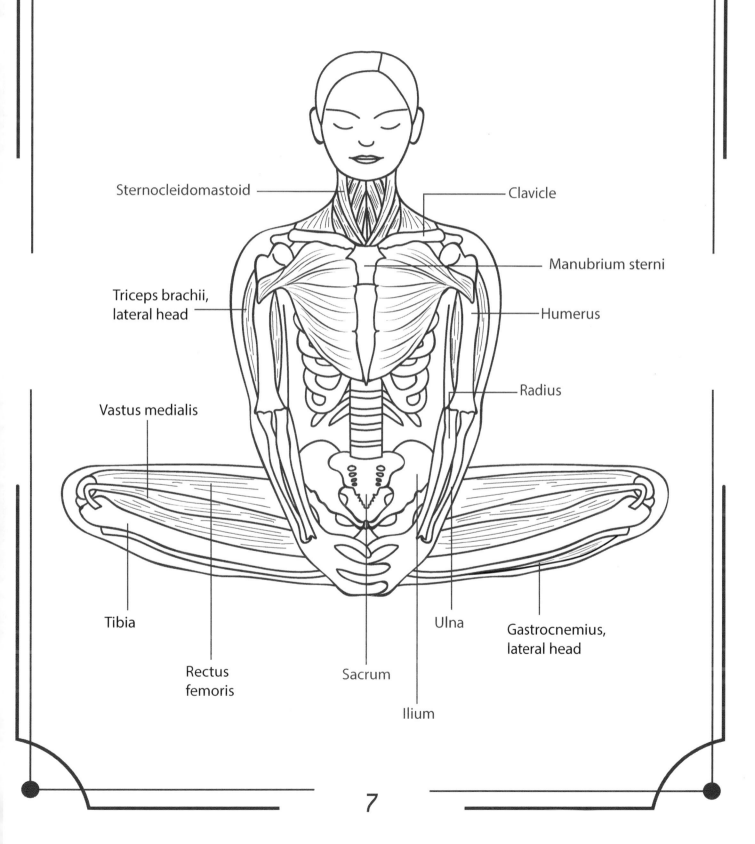

Sternocleidomastoid

Clavicle

Manubrium sterni

Triceps brachii, lateral head

Humerus

Vastus medialis

Radius

Tibia

Ulna

Gastrocnemius, lateral head

Rectus femoris

Sacrum

Ilium

Bow Pose
Dhanurāsana

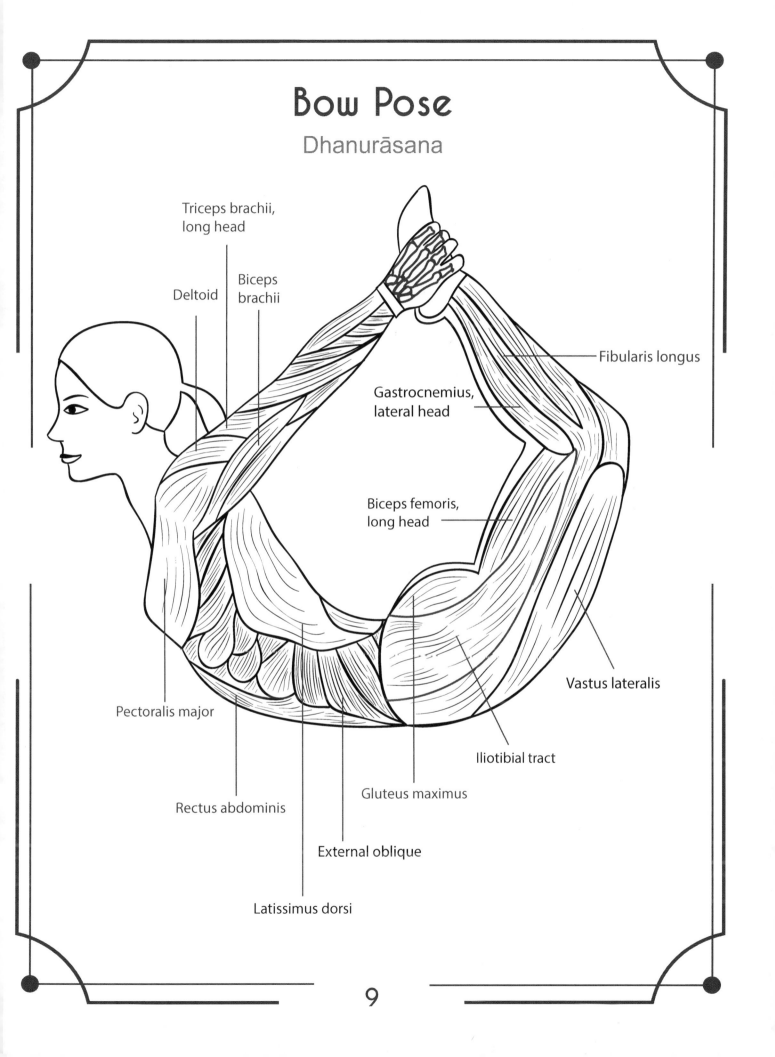

Triceps brachii, long head

Deltoid

Biceps brachii

Fibularis longus

Gastrocnemius, lateral head

Biceps femoris, long head

Vastus lateralis

Pectoralis major

Iliotibial tract

Rectus abdominis

Gluteus maximus

External oblique

Latissimus dorsi

Bridge Pose

Setu Bandha Sarvāṅgāsana

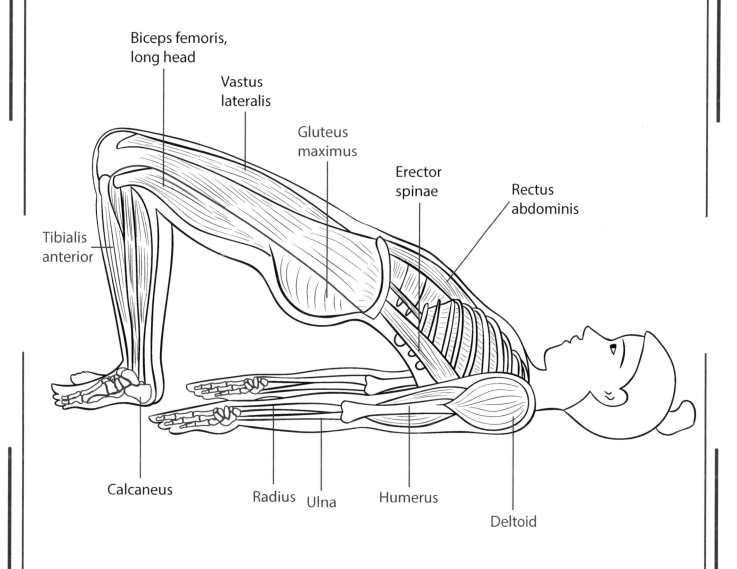

Biceps femoris,
long head

Vastus
lateralis

Gluteus
maximus

Erector
spinae

Rectus
abdominis

Tibialis
anterior

Calcaneus

Radius

Ulna

Humerus

Deltoid

Camel Pose

Uṣṭrāsana

Pectoralis major

Deltoid

Latissimus dorsi

Iliotibial tract

Triceps brachii, long head

Biceps brachii

Gluteus maximus

Biceps femoris

Gastrocnemius

Vastus lateralis

Soleus

Chair Pose
Utkaṭāsana

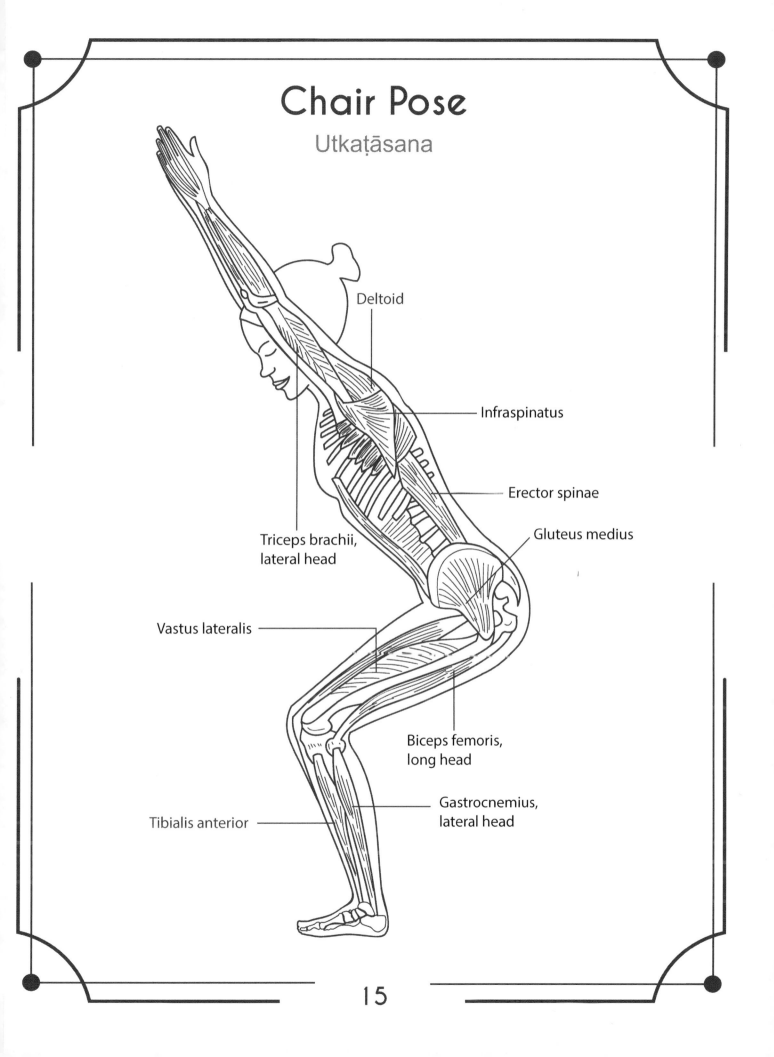

Deltoid

Infraspinatus

Erector spinae

Gluteus medius

Triceps brachii,
lateral head

Vastus lateralis

Biceps femoris,
long head

Gastrocnemius,
lateral head

Tibialis anterior

Child's Pose

Bālāsana

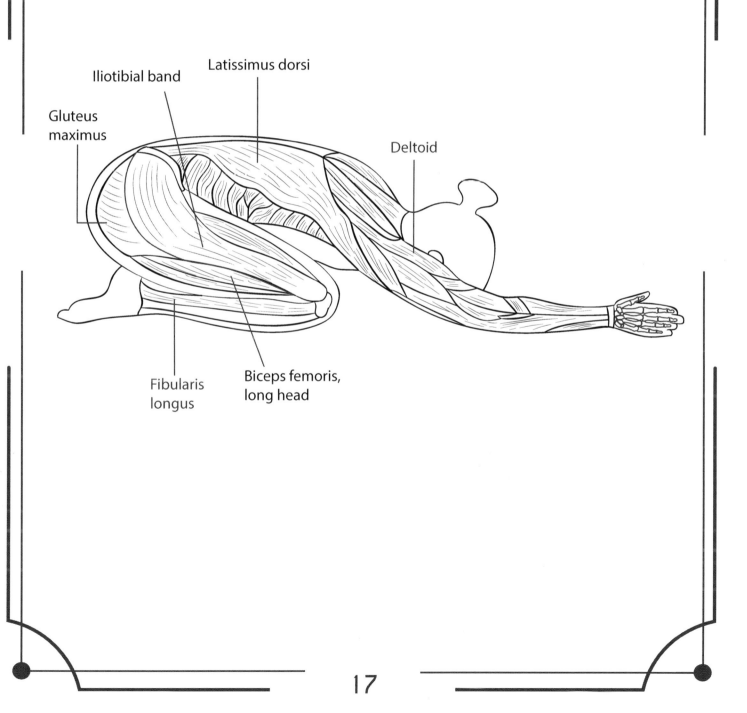

Gluteus maximus

Iliotibial band

Latissimus dorsi

Deltoid

Fibularis longus

Biceps femoris, long head

Cobra Pose
Bhujaṅgāsana

Deltoid

Triceps
brachii

Gluteus
maximus

Biceps
femoris,
long head

Gastrocnemius,
lateral head

Fibularis longus

Vastus lateralis

Iliotibial
tract

Boat Pose
Nāvāsana

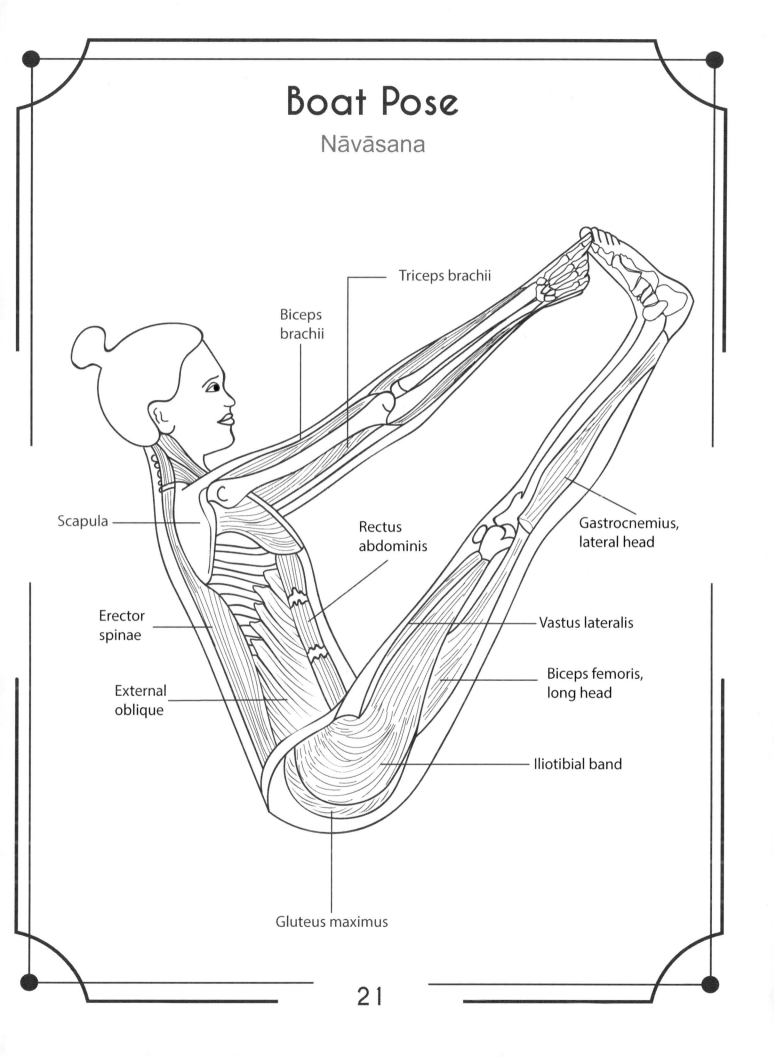

Triceps brachii

Biceps brachii

Scapula

Rectus abdominis

Erector spinae

Gastrocnemius, lateral head

Vastus lateralis

External oblique

Biceps femoris, long head

Iliotibial band

Gluteus maximus

Crow Pose

Bakāsana

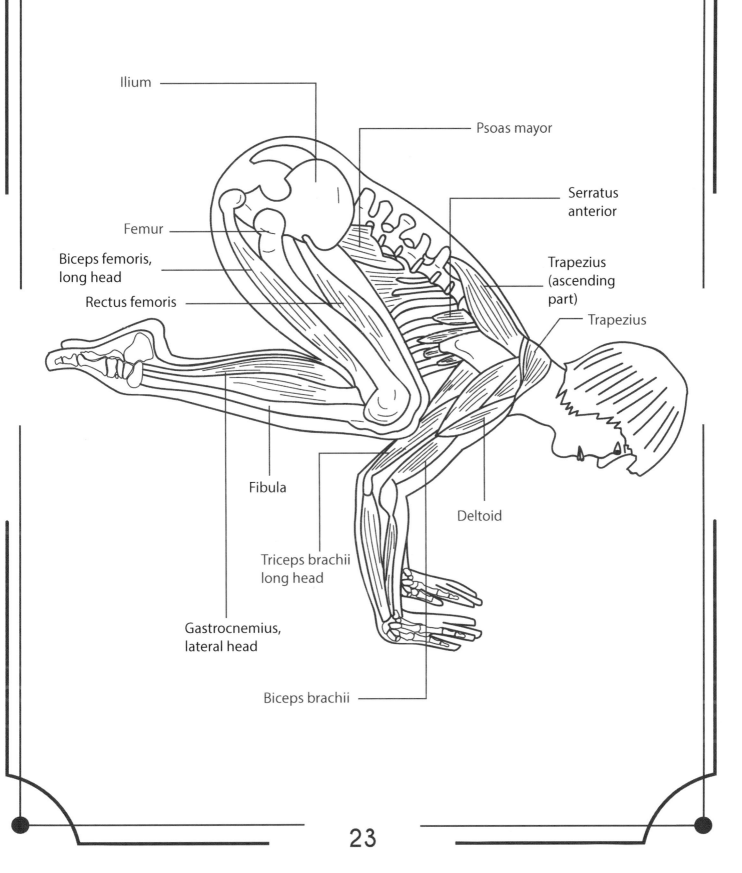

Ilium

Psoas mayor

Serratus anterior

Femur

Biceps femoris, long head

Trapezius (ascending part)

Rectus femoris

Trapezius

Fibula

Deltoid

Triceps brachii long head

Gastrocnemius, lateral head

Biceps brachii

Downward Dog Pose

Adho Mukha Śvānāsana

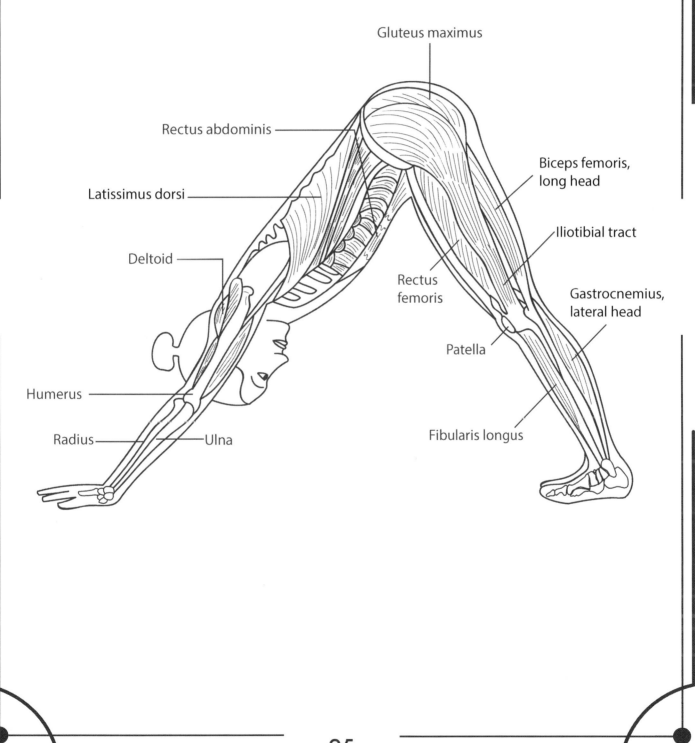

Gluteus maximus

Rectus abdominis

Latissimus dorsi

Biceps femoris,
long head

Iliotibial tract

Deltoid

Rectus
femoris

Gastrocnemius,
lateral head

Patella

Humerus

Radius — Ulna

Fibularis longus

Eagle Pose

Garuḍāsana

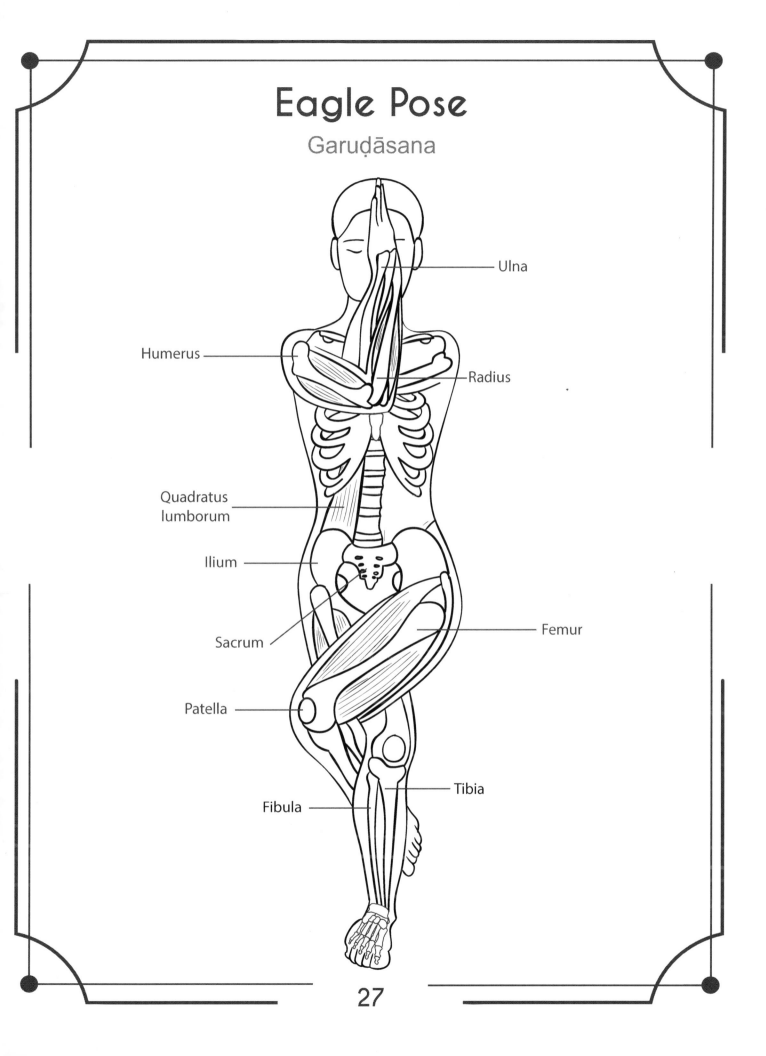

Ulna

Humerus

Radius

Quadratus
lumborum

Ilium

Sacrum

Femur

Patella

Tibia

Fibula

Extended Puppy Pose
Uttāna Shishosana

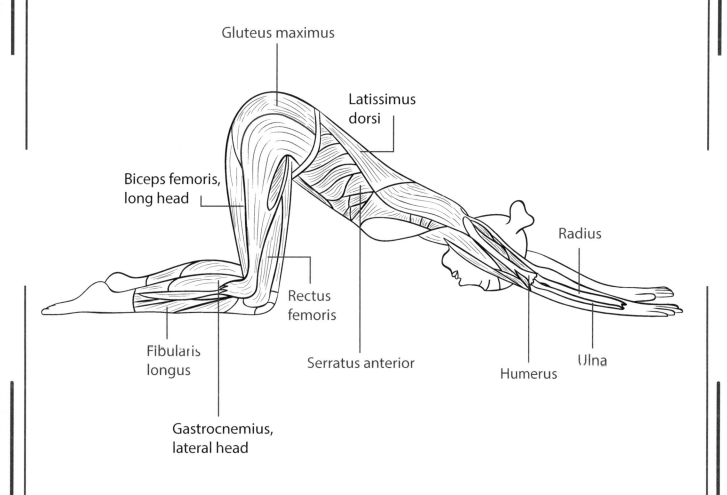

Gluteus maximus

Latissimus dorsi

Biceps femoris, long head

Rectus femoris

Radius

Fibularis longus

Serratus anterior

Humerus

Ulna

Gastrocnemius, lateral head

Extended Side Angle Pose

Utthita Páršvakónásana

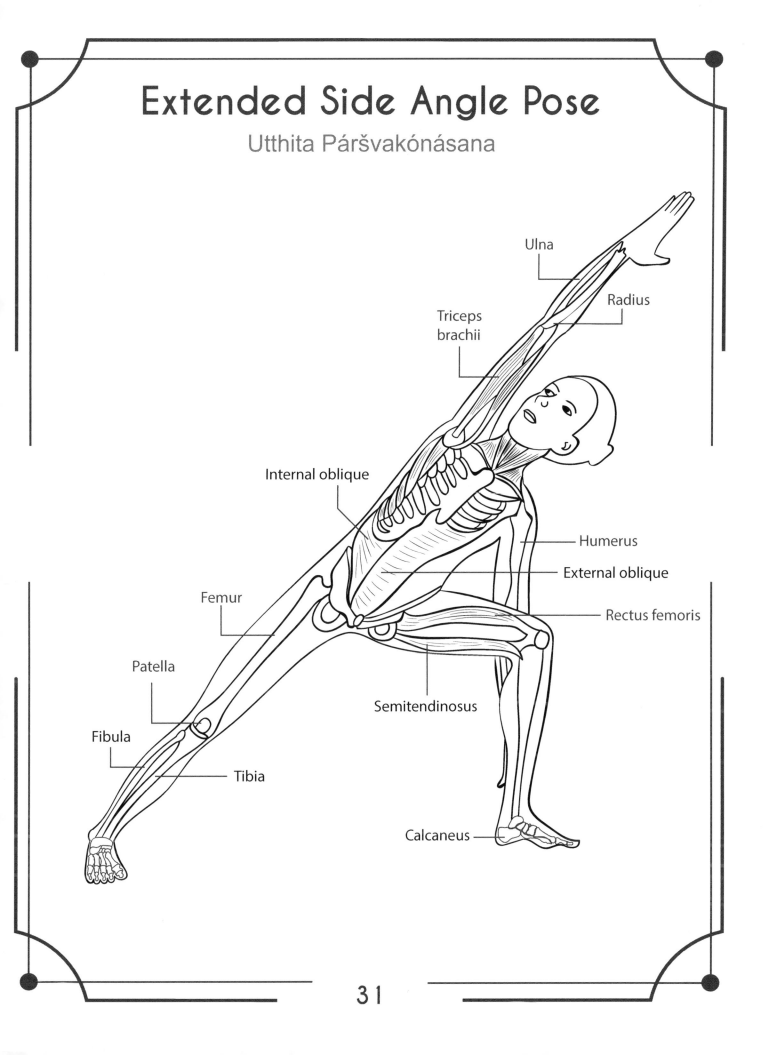

Ulna

Triceps
brachii

Radius

Internal oblique

Humerus

External oblique

Rectus femoris

Femur

Patella

Semitendinosus

Fibula

Tibia

Calcaneus

Frog's Pose

Mandukāsana

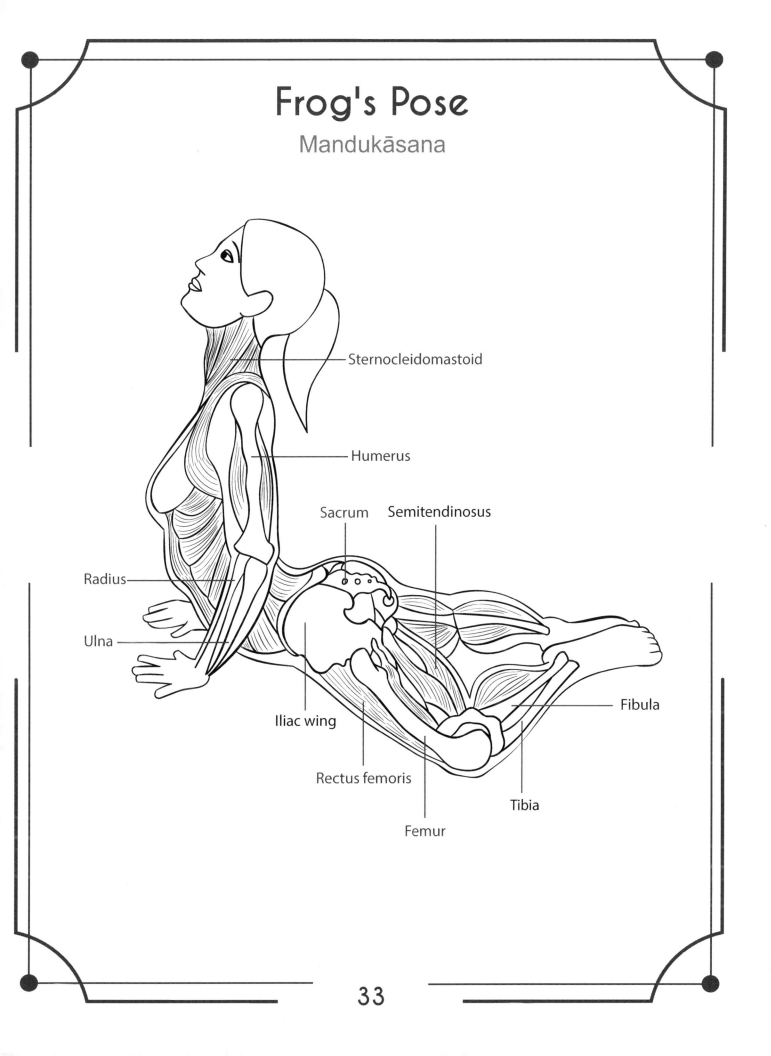

Sternocleidomastoid

Humerus

Sacrum   Semitendinosus

Radius

Ulna

Iliac wing

Fibula

Rectus femoris

Tibia

Femur

Half Lord of the Fishes Pose

Ardha Matsyendrāsana

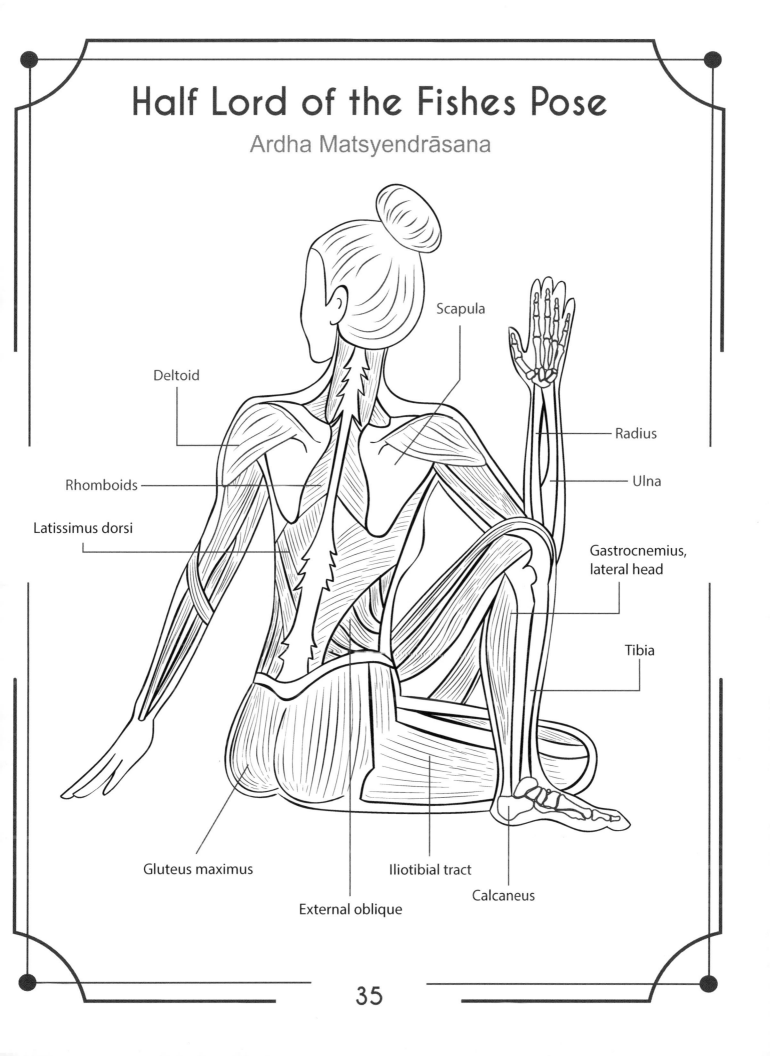

Scapula

Deltoid

Rhomboids

Latissimus dorsi

Radius

Ulna

Gastrocnemius, lateral head

Tibia

Gluteus maximus

Iliotibial tract

Calcaneus

External oblique

Hand To Big Toe Pose

Utthita Hasta Pādāngusthāsana

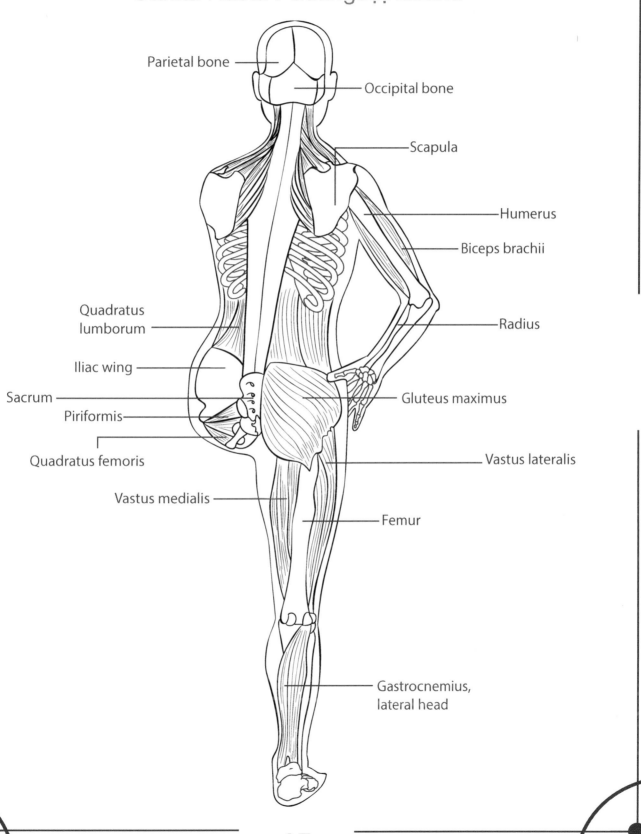

Parietal bone

Occipital bone

Scapula

Humerus

Biceps brachii

Quadratus lumborum

Radius

Iliac wing

Sacrum

Gluteus maximus

Piriformis

Quadratus femoris

Vastus lateralis

Vastus medialis

Femur

Gastrocnemius, lateral head

Handstand Pose

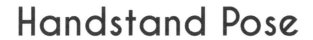

Adho Mukha Vrkṣāsana

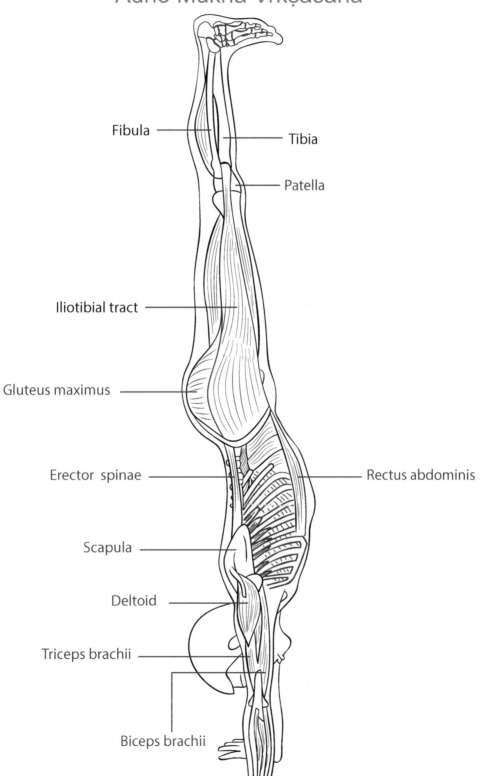

Fibula

Tibia

Patella

Iliotibial tract

Gluteus maximus

Erector spinae

Rectus abdominis

Scapula

Deltoid

Triceps brachii

Biceps brachii

Headstand Pose

Sālamba Śīrṣāsana

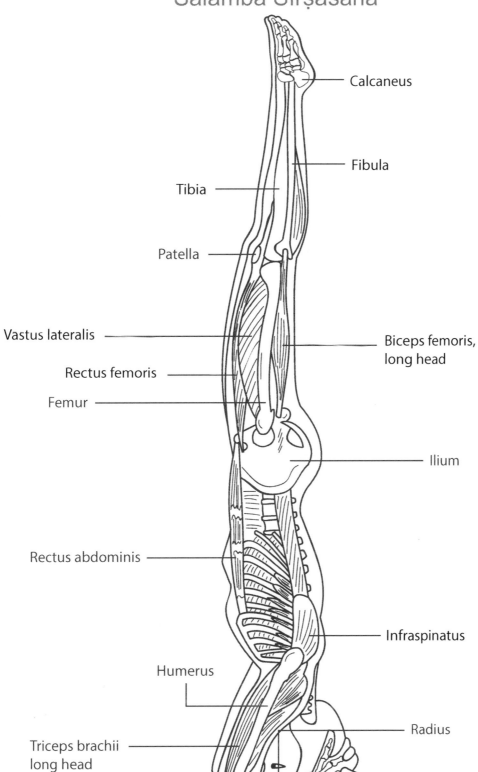

Calcaneus

Fibula

Tibia

Patella

Vastus lateralis

Rectus femoris

Femur

Biceps femoris, long head

Ilium

Rectus abdominis

Infraspinatus

Humerus

Radius

Triceps brachii long head

Ulna

Hero's Pose
Vīrāsana

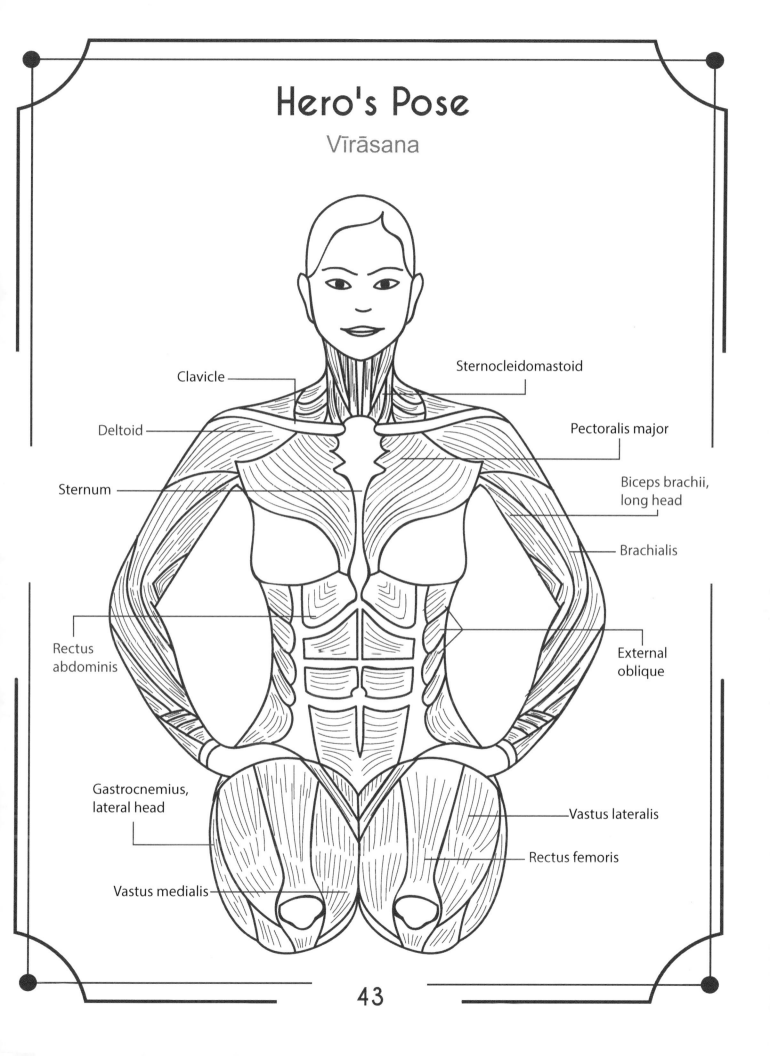

Clavicle

Sternocleidomastoid

Deltoid

Pectoralis major

Sternum

Biceps brachii, long head

Brachialis

Rectus abdominis

External oblique

Gastrocnemius, lateral head

Vastus lateralis

Rectus femoris

Vastus medialis

King Dancer Pose
Naṭarājāsana

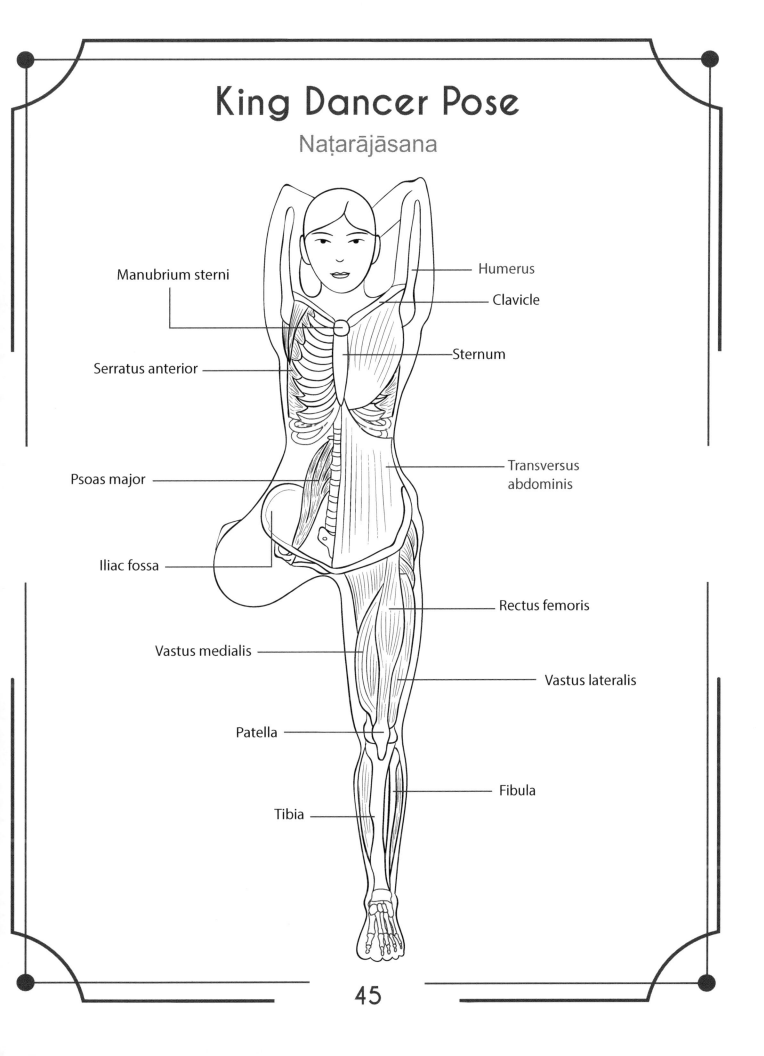

Manubrium sterni

Humerus

Clavicle

Sternum

Serratus anterior

Transversus
abdominis

Psoas major

Iliac fossa

Rectus femoris

Vastus medialis

Vastus lateralis

Patella

Fibula

Tibia

Legs Up The Wall Pose

Viparīta Karaṇī

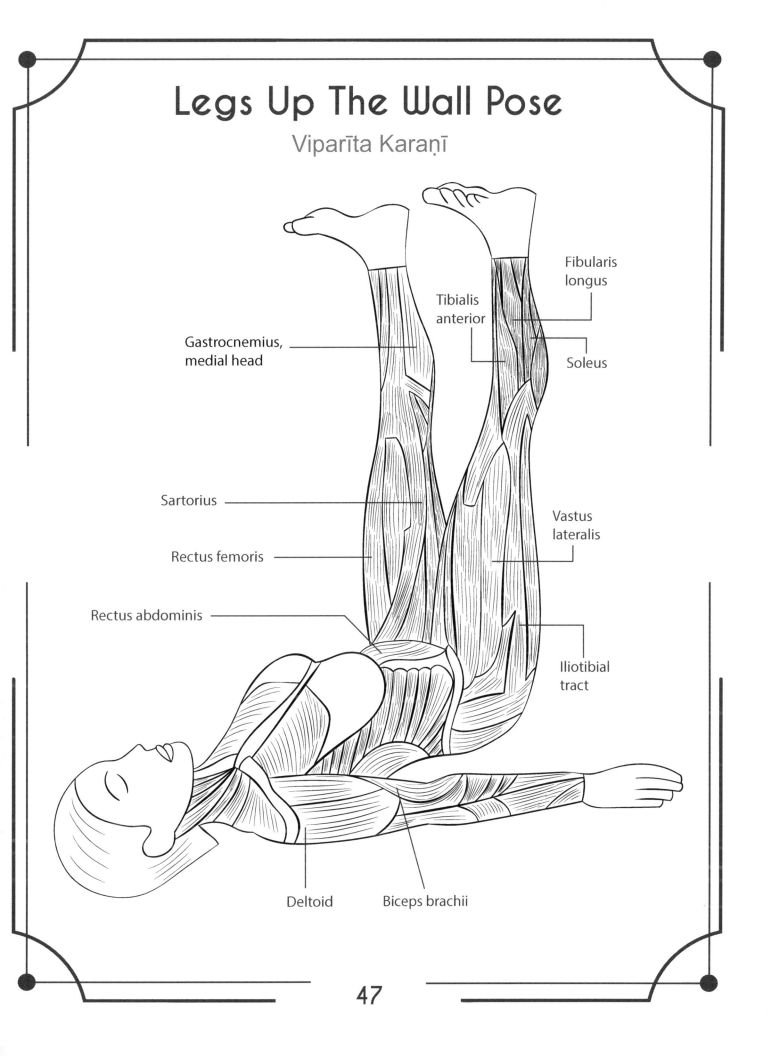

Fibularis longus

Tibialis anterior

Soleus

Gastrocnemius, medial head

Sartorius

Vastus lateralis

Rectus femoris

Rectus abdominis

Iliotibial tract

Deltoid

Biceps brachii

Mountain Pose

Tāḍāsana

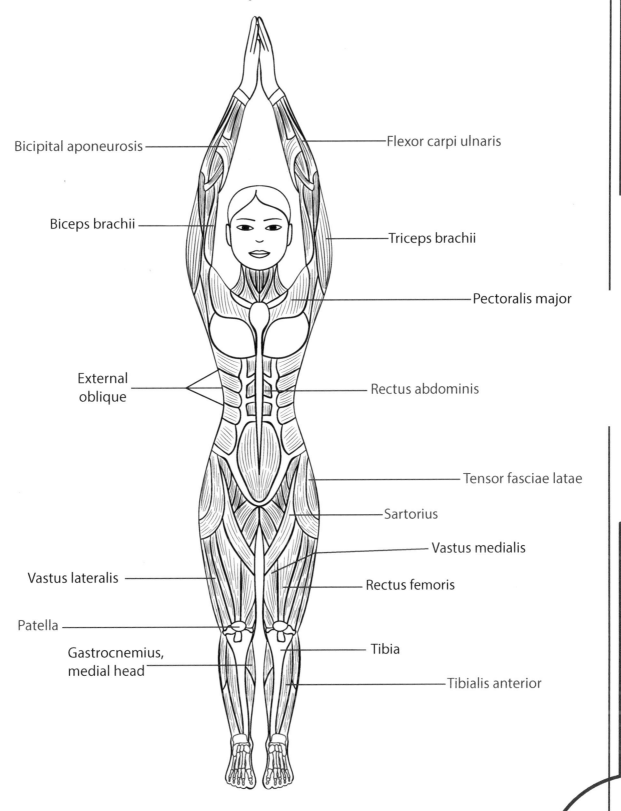

Bicipital aponeurosis

Flexor carpi ulnaris

Biceps brachii

Triceps brachii

Pectoralis major

External oblique

Rectus abdominis

Tensor fasciae latae

Sartorius

Vastus medialis

Vastus lateralis

Rectus femoris

Patella

Tibia

Gastrocnemius, medial head

Tibialis anterior

Peacock Pose

Mayūrāsana

Gluteus
maximus

Tibia

Iliotibial
tract

Erector
spinae

Fibula

Scapula

Vastus
lateralis

Patella

Humerus

Radius

Ulna

4-Limbed Staff Pose
Chaturanga Dandasana

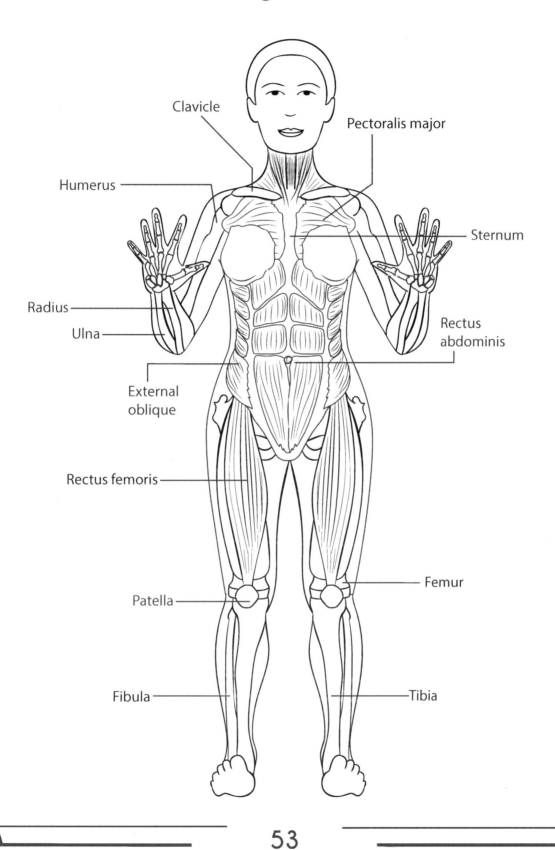

Clavicle

Pectoralis major

Humerus

Sternum

Radius

Ulna

Rectus abdominis

External oblique

Rectus femoris

Femur

Patella

Fibula

Tibia

Plow Pose

Halasana

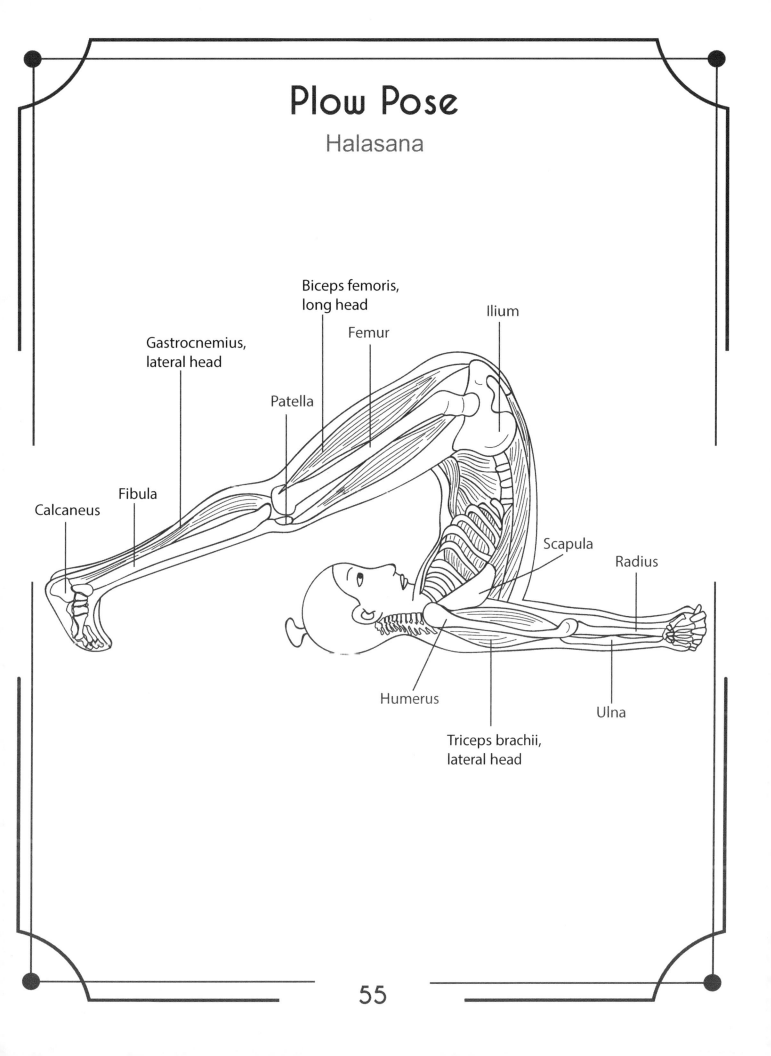

Biceps femoris, long head

Gastrocnemius, lateral head

Ilium

Femur

Patella

Fibula

Calcaneus

Scapula

Radius

Humerus

Ulna

Triceps brachii, lateral head

Pyramid Pose
Parsvottanasana

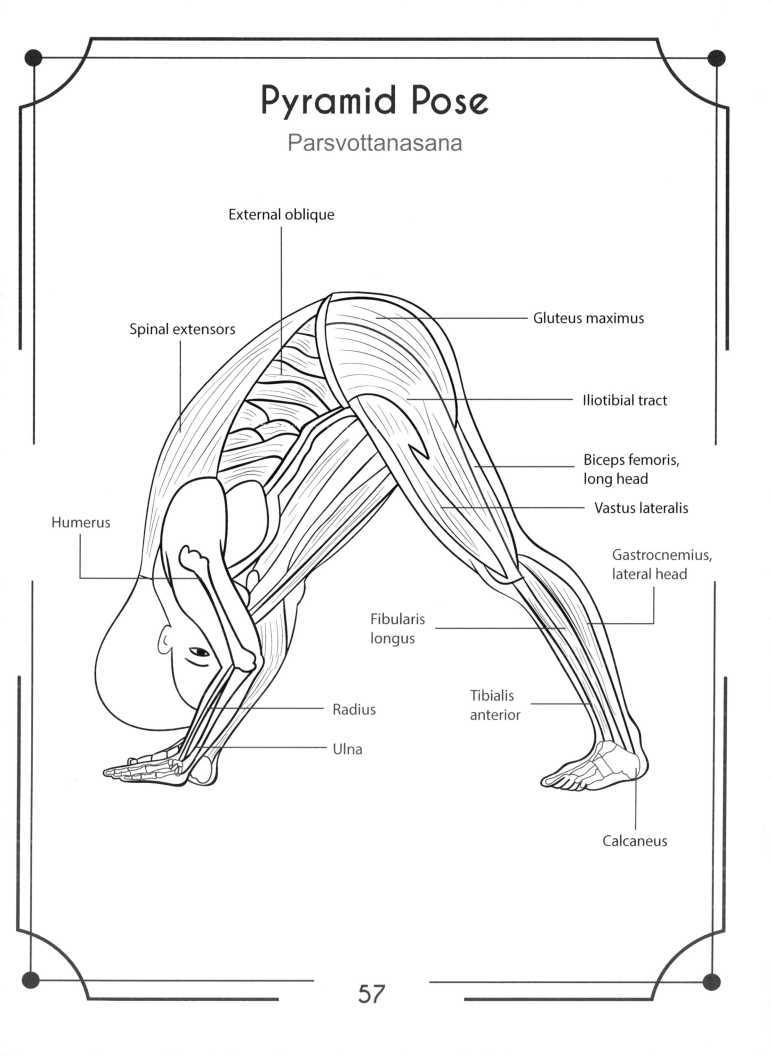

External oblique

Spinal extensors

Gluteus maximus

Iliotibial tract

Biceps femoris, long head

Vastus lateralis

Humerus

Gastrocnemius, lateral head

Fibularis longus

Radius

Tibialis anterior

Ulna

Calcaneus

Reclined Hero Pose

Supta Virasana

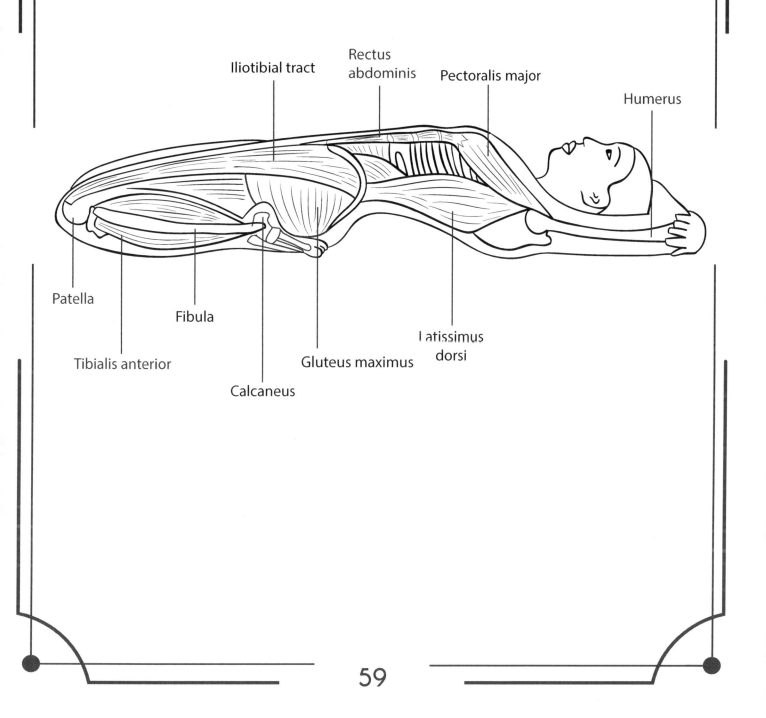

Iliotibial tract

Rectus abdominis

Pectoralis major

Humerus

Patella

Fibula

Tibialis anterior

Calcaneus

Gluteus maximus

Latissimus dorsi

Reverse Prayer Pose

Pashchima Namaskarasana

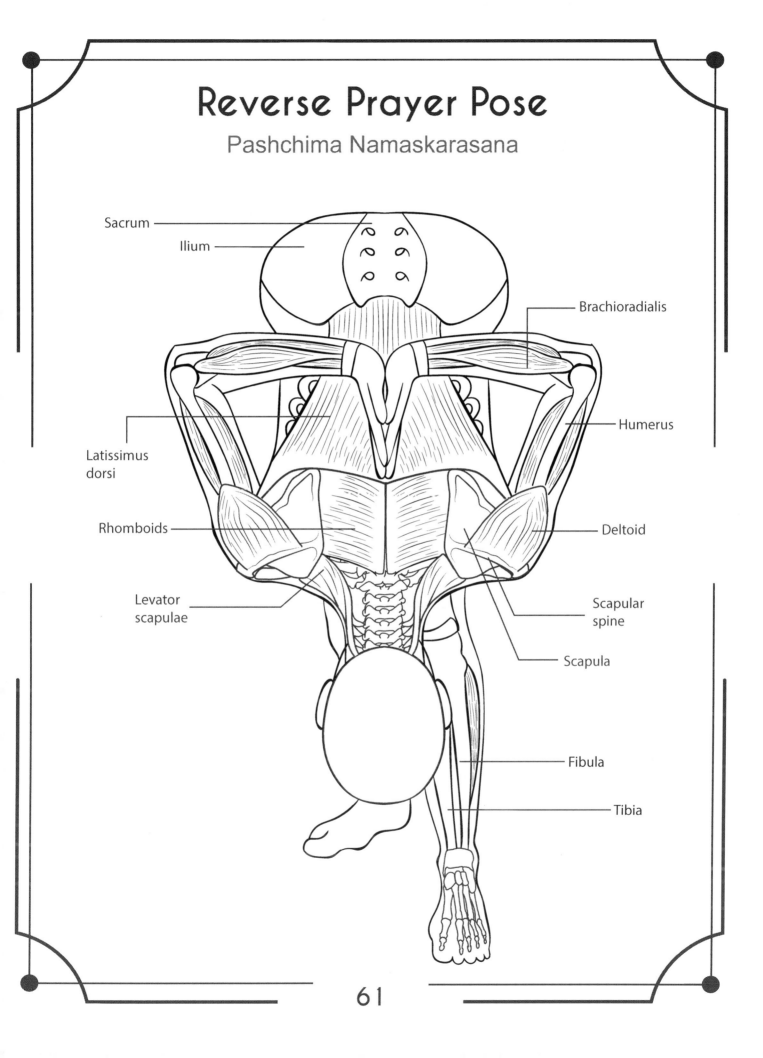

Sacrum

Ilium

Brachioradialis

Humerus

Latissimus dorsi

Rhomboids

Deltoid

Levator scapulae

Scapular spine

Scapula

Fibula

Tibia

Reverse Table Top Pose

Ardha Pūrvottānāsana

Spine

Deltoid

Rib cage

Scapula

Vastus lateralis

Gluteus medius

Iliotibial tract

Triceps brachii, lateral head

Biceps femoris, long head

Gluteus maximus

Radius

Ulna

Fibula

Calcaneus

Tibia

Revolved Side Angle Pose

Parivṛtta Párśvakónásana

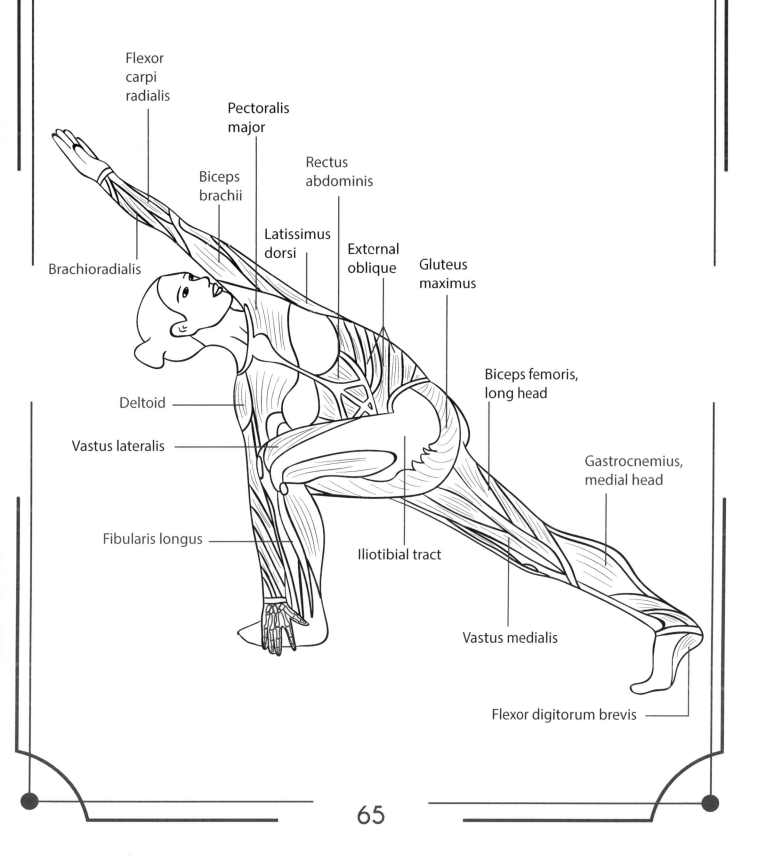

- Flexor carpi radialis
- Pectoralis major
- Rectus abdominis
- Biceps brachii
- Latissimus dorsi
- External oblique
- Gluteus maximus
- Brachioradialis
- Biceps femoris, long head
- Deltoid
- Vastus lateralis
- Gastrocnemius, medial head
- Fibularis longus
- Iliotibial tract
- Vastus medialis
- Flexor digitorum brevis

Revolved Triangle Pose
Parivṛtta Trikoṇāsana

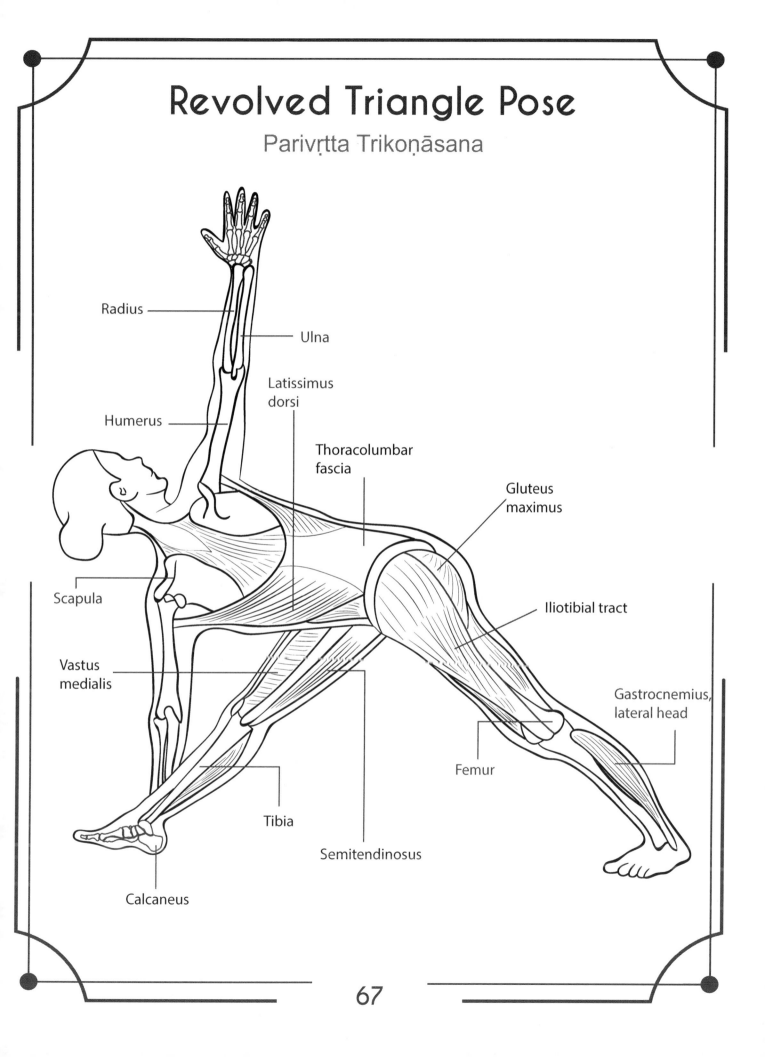

Radius

Ulna

Latissimus dorsi

Humerus

Thoracolumbar fascia

Gluteus maximus

Scapula

Iliotibial tract

Vastus medialis

Gastrocnemius, lateral head

Femur

Tibia

Semitendinosus

Calcaneus

Seated Forward Fold Pose

Paścimottānāsana

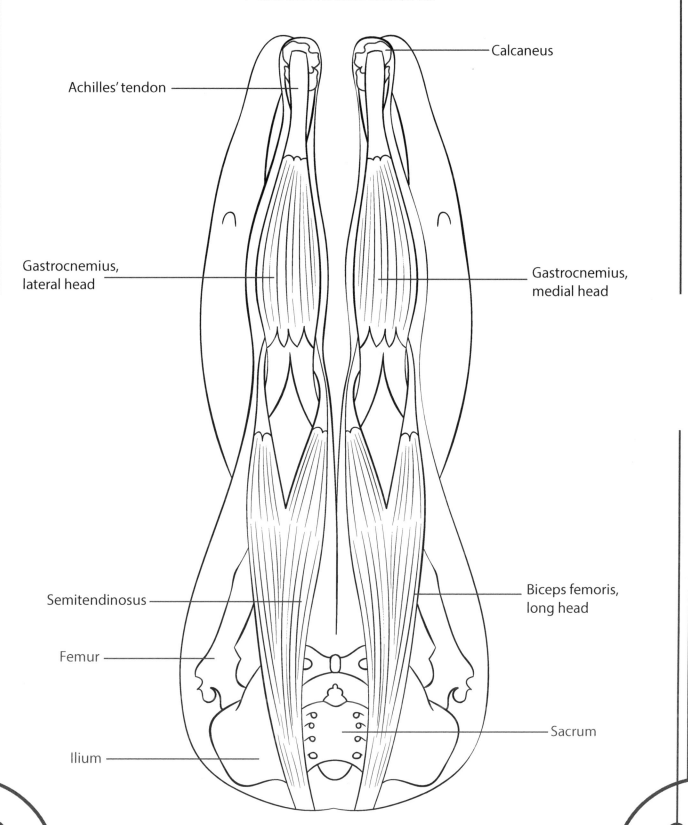

Calcaneus

Achilles' tendon

Gastrocnemius,
lateral head

Gastrocnemius,
medial head

Semitendinosus

Biceps femoris,
long head

Femur

Ilium

Sacrum

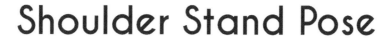

Shoulder Stand Pose
Sālamba Sarvāṅgāsana

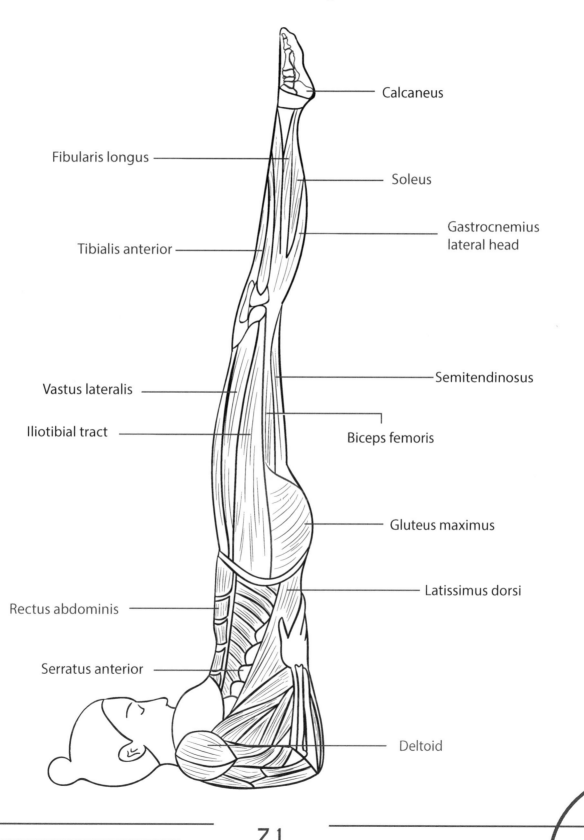

Calcaneus

Fibularis longus

Soleus

Gastrocnemius
lateral head

Tibialis anterior

Semitendinosus

Vastus lateralis

Iliotibial tract

Biceps femoris

Gluteus maximus

Latissimus dorsi

Rectus abdominis

Serratus anterior

Deltoid

Side Crow Pose

Pārśva Bakāsana

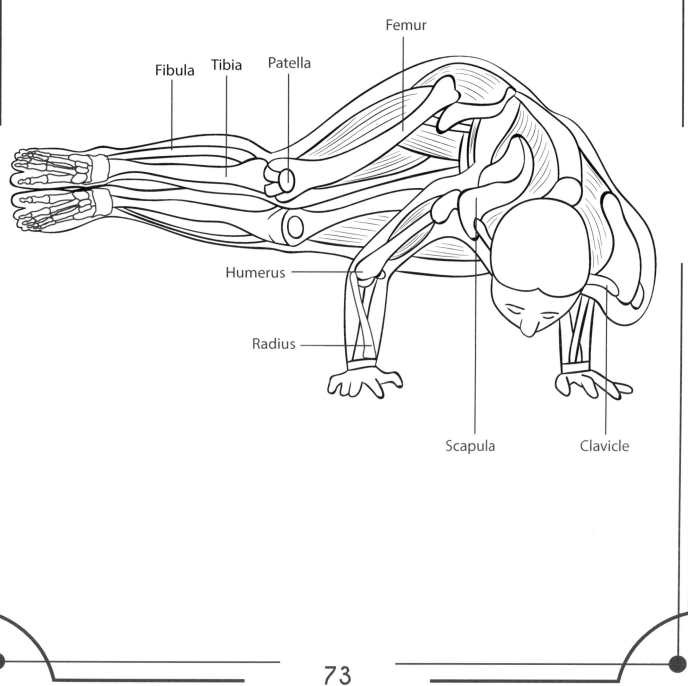

Femur

Fibula   Tibia   Patella

Humerus

Radius

Scapula   Clavicle

Splits Pose

Hanumanásana

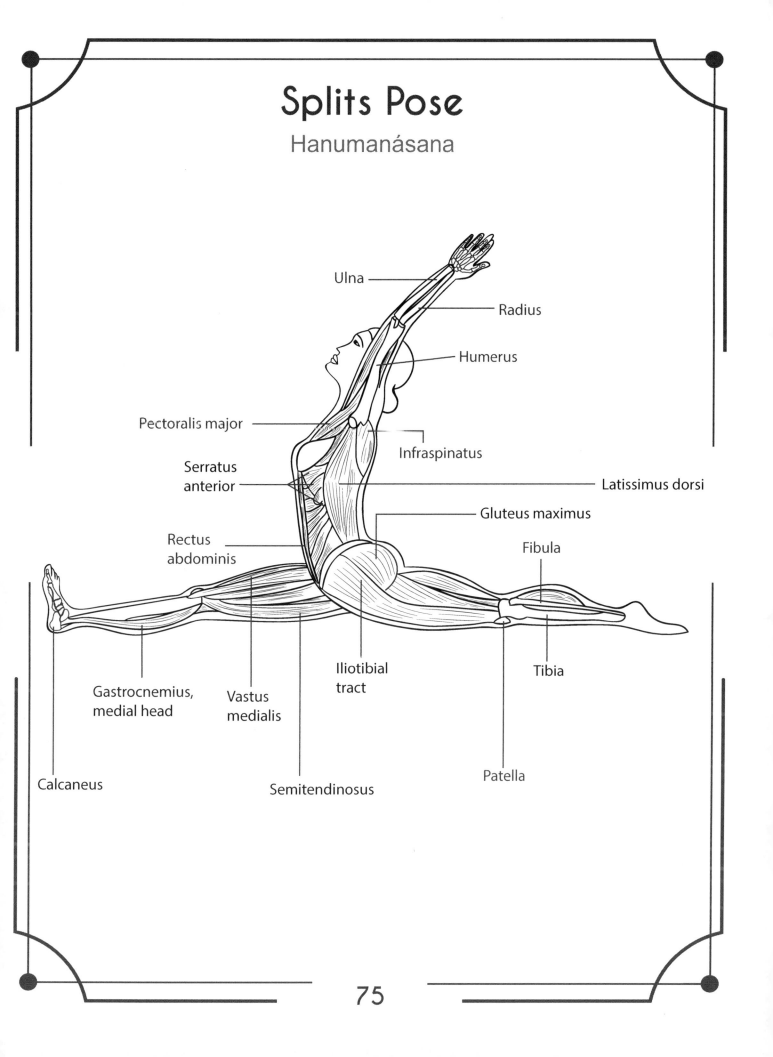

Ulna

Radius

Humerus

Pectoralis major

Infraspinatus

Serratus anterior

Latissimus dorsi

Gluteus maximus

Rectus abdominis

Fibula

Iliotibial tract

Tibia

Gastrocnemius, medial head

Vastus medialis

Calcaneus

Semitendinosus

Patella

Garland Pose

Mālāsana

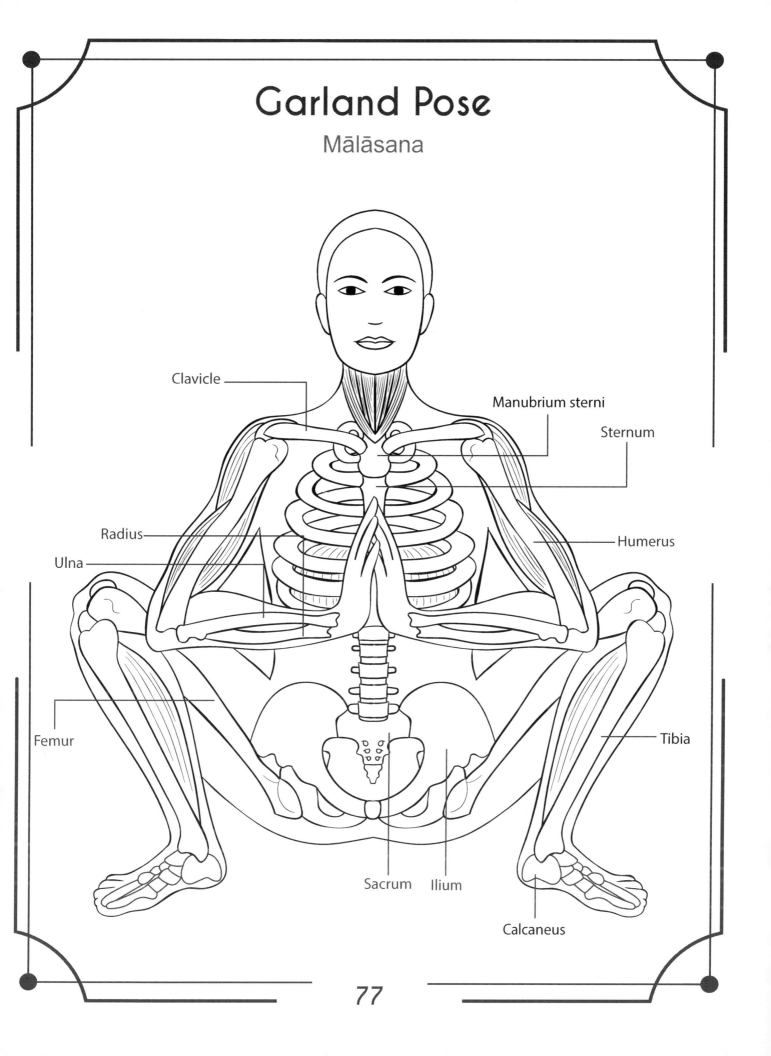

Clavicle

Manubrium sterni

Sternum

Radius

Humerus

Ulna

Femur

Tibia

Sacrum   Ilium

Calcaneus

Staff Pose

Daṇḍāsana

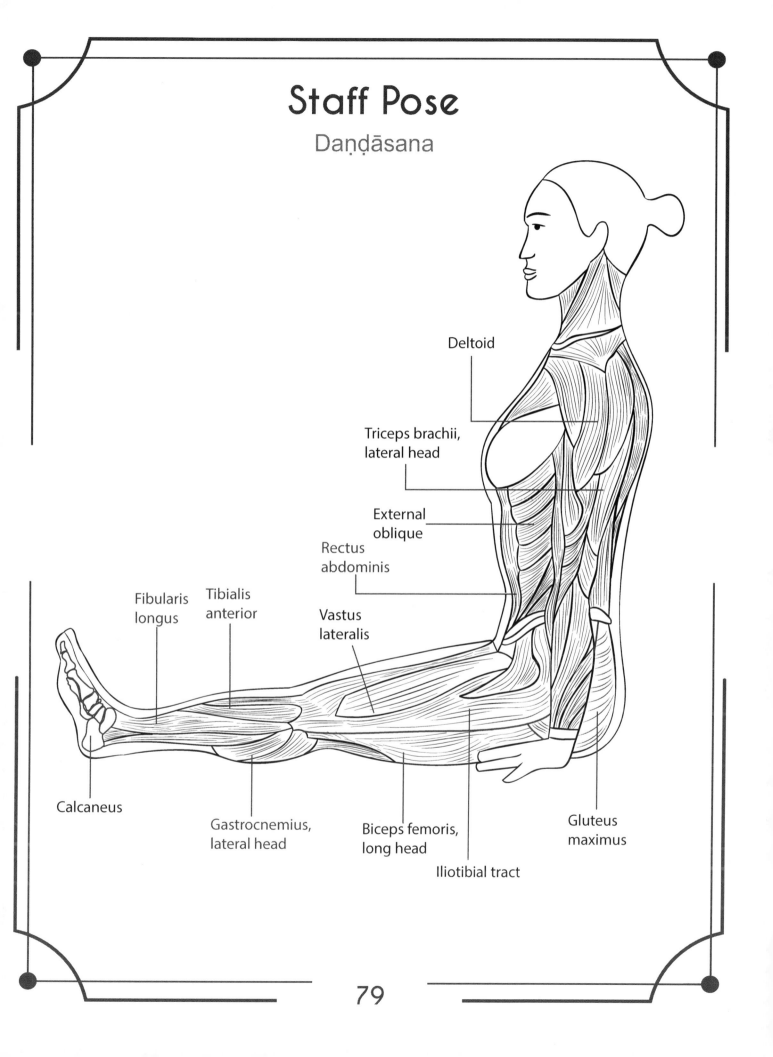

Deltoid

Triceps brachii, lateral head

External oblique

Rectus abdominis

Fibularis longus

Tibialis anterior

Vastus lateralis

Calcaneus

Gastrocnemius, lateral head

Biceps femoris, long head

Iliotibial tract

Gluteus maximus

Standing Forward Fold Pose

Uttānasana

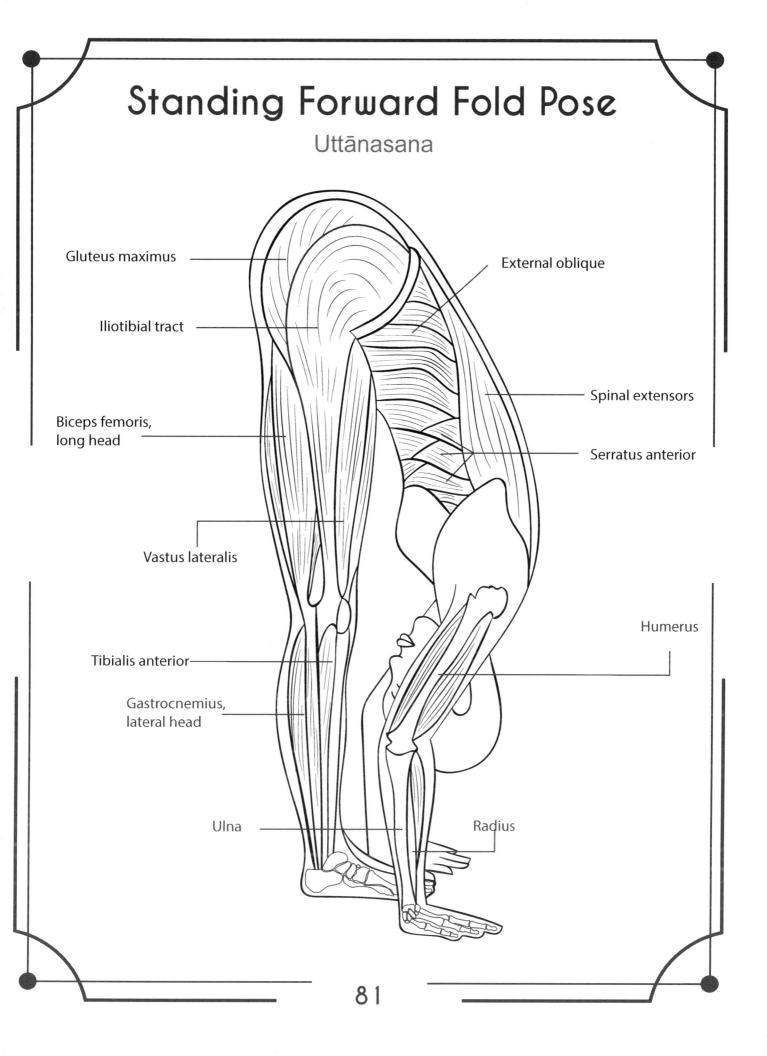

Gluteus maximus

Iliotibial tract

Biceps femoris, long head

Vastus lateralis

Tibialis anterior

Gastrocnemius, lateral head

Ulna

External oblique

Spinal extensors

Serratus anterior

Humerus

Radius

Tree Pose

Vrkṣāsana

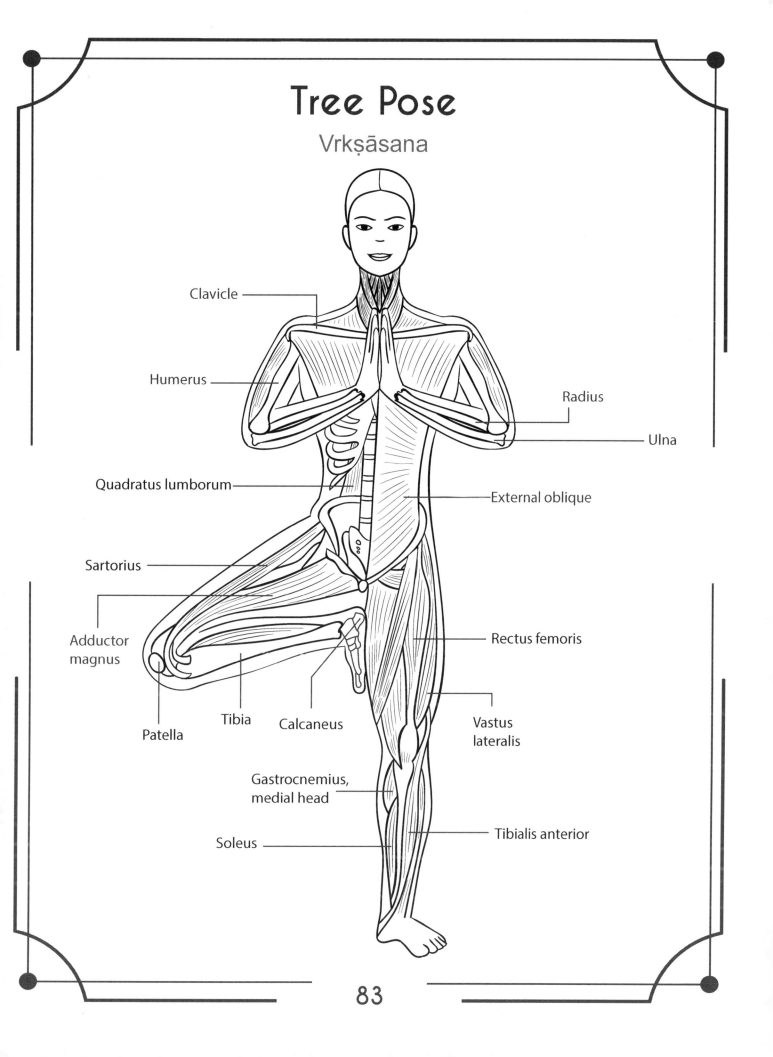

Clavicle

Humerus

Radius

Ulna

Quadratus lumborum

External oblique

Sartorius

Rectus femoris

Adductor
magnus

Tibia

Calcaneus

Vastus
lateralis

Patella

Gastrocnemius,
medial head

Tibialis anterior

Soleus

Bound Revolved Side Angle

Baddha Parivṛtta Parśvakoṇāsana

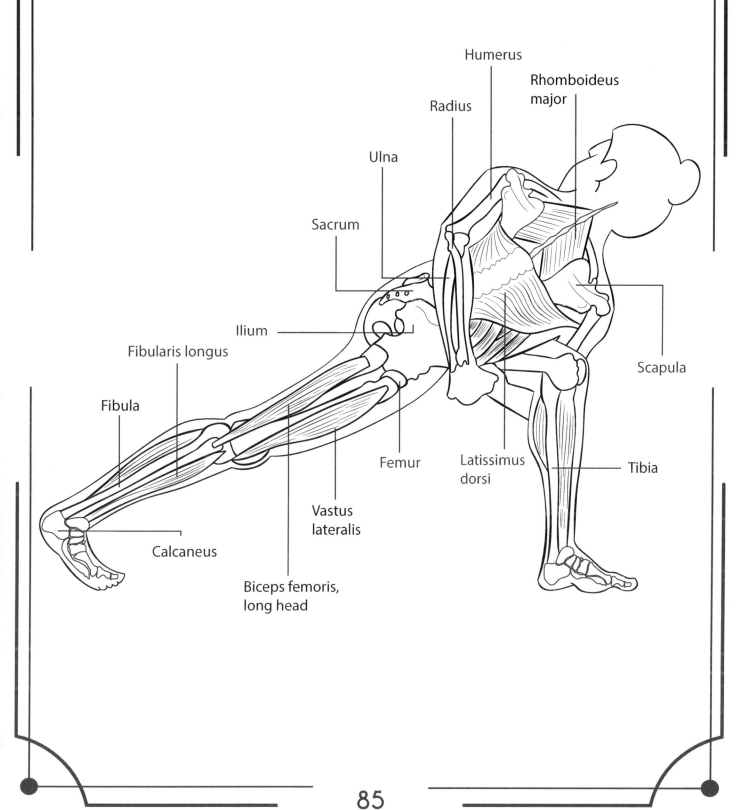

Humerus

Rhomboideus major

Radius

Ulna

Sacrum

Ilium

Fibularis longus

Fibula

Scapula

Femur

Latissimus dorsi

Tibia

Vastus lateralis

Calcaneus

Biceps femoris, long head

Upward Facing Dog Pose

Urdhva mukha śvānāsana

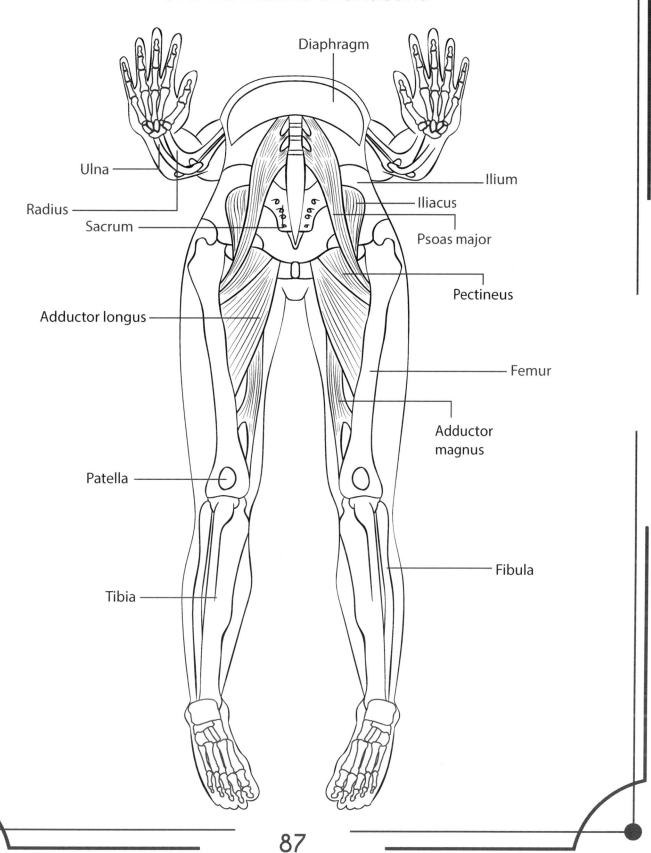

Diaphragm

Ulna

Radius

Sacrum

Ilium

Iliacus

Psoas major

Pectineus

Adductor longus

Femur

Adductor magnus

Patella

Fibula

Tibia

Upward Plank Pose

Pūrvottānāsana

Rectus
abdominis

Iliotibial tract

Vastus
lateralis

Gastrocnemius,
lateral head

Scapula

Triceps brachii

Gluteus
maximus

Humerus

Biceps femoris,
long head

Ulna

Calcaneus

Warrior I Pose

Virabhadrāsana I

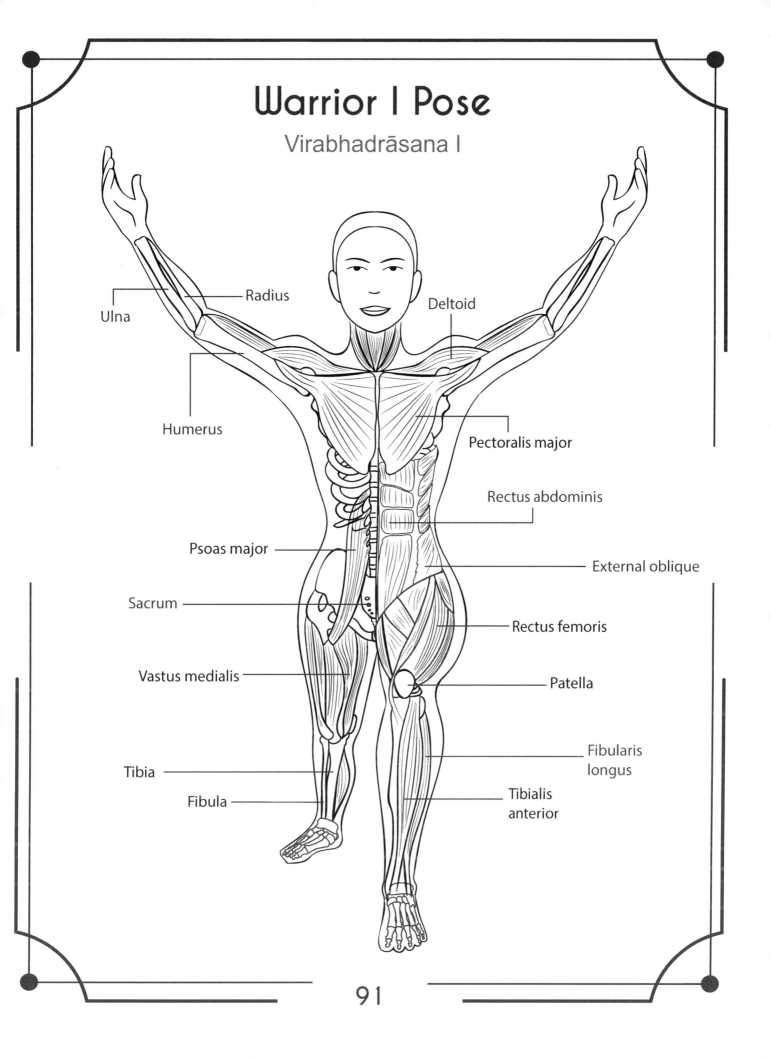

Radius

Ulna

Deltoid

Humerus

Pectoralis major

Rectus abdominis

Psoas major

External oblique

Sacrum

Rectus femoris

Vastus medialis

Patella

Tibia

Fibularis longus

Fibula

Tibialis anterior

Warrior II Pose

Virabhadrāsana II

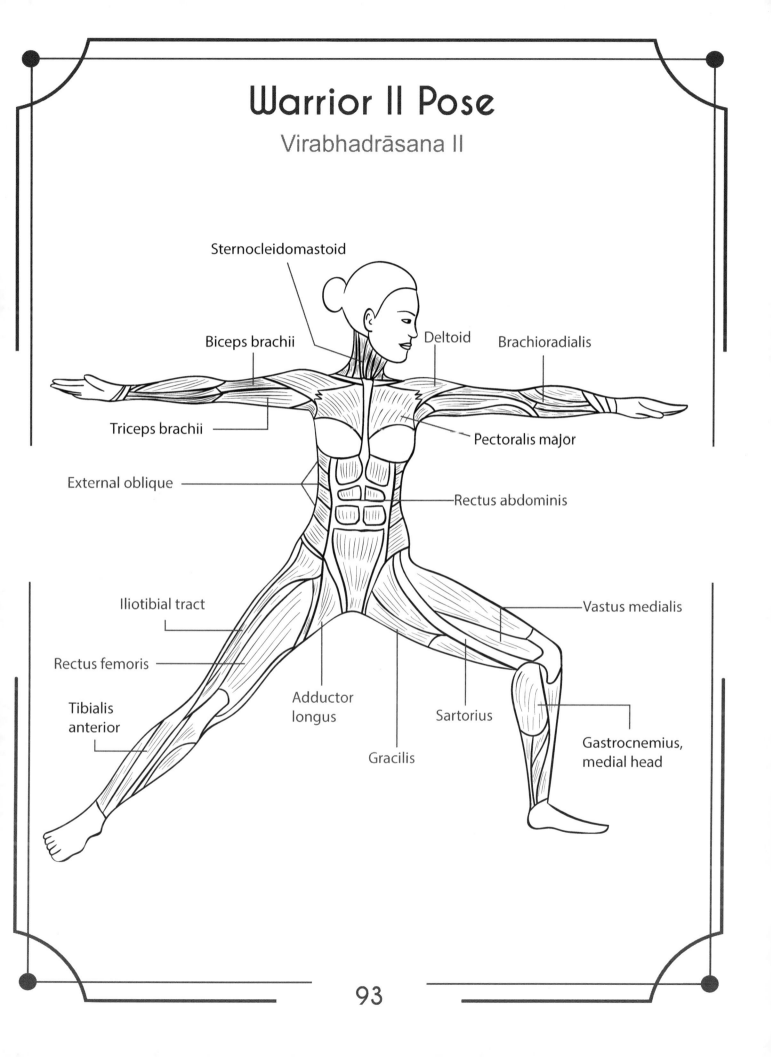

Sternocleidomastoid

Biceps brachii

Deltoid

Brachioradialis

Triceps brachii

Pectoralis major

External oblique

Rectus abdominis

Iliotibial tract

Vastus medialis

Rectus femoris

Adductor longus

Sartorius

Tibialis anterior

Gracilis

Gastrocnemius, medial head

Warrior III Pose

Virabhadrāsana III

Ulna

Scapula

External oblique

Gluteus maximus

Femur

Gastrocnemius, medial head

Tibia

Humerus

Rectus femoris

Patella

Biceps femoris, long head

Iliotibial tract

Fibula

Gastrocnemius, lateral head

Calcaneus

Wheel Pose
Chakrāsana

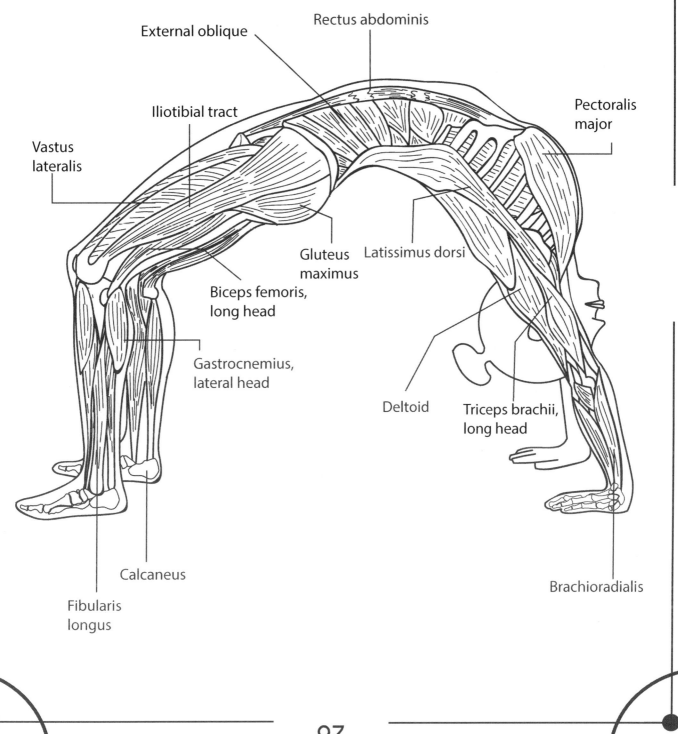

External oblique

Rectus abdominis

Iliotibial tract

Pectoralis major

Vastus lateralis

Gluteus maximus

Latissimus dorsi

Biceps femoris, long head

Gastrocnemius, lateral head

Deltoid

Triceps brachii, long head

Calcaneus

Brachioradialis

Fibularis longus

Wide-Legged Forward Fold

Prasārita Pādottānāsana

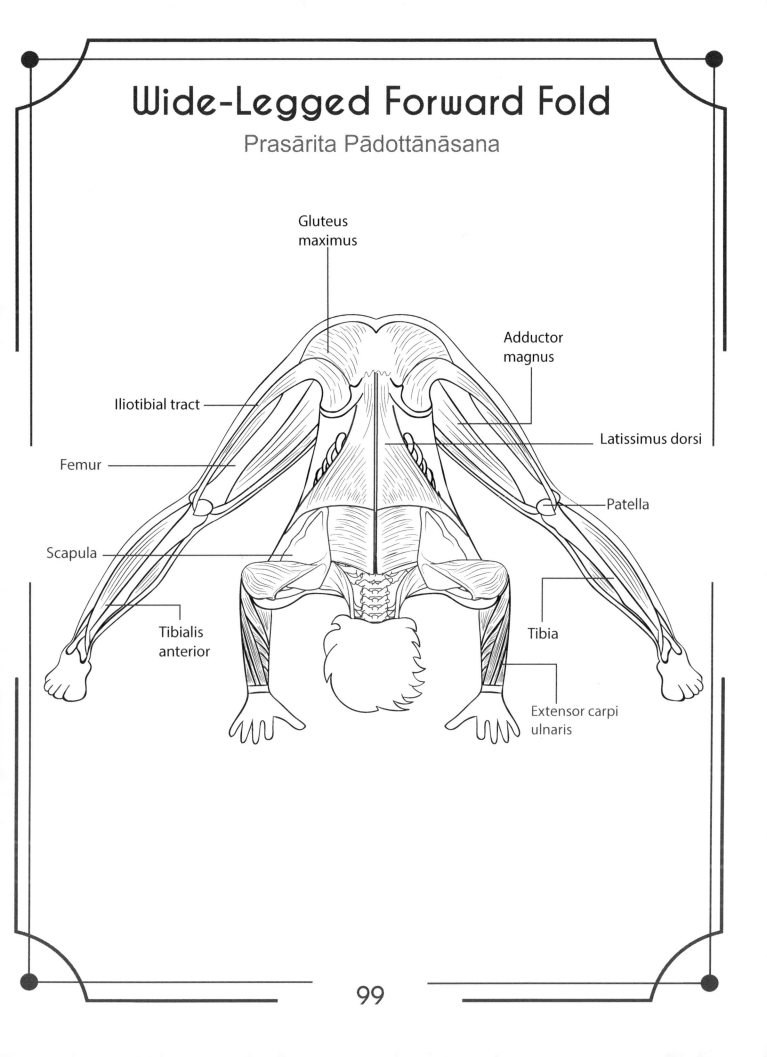

Gluteus maximus

Adductor magnus

Iliotibial tract

Latissimus dorsi

Femur

Patella

Scapula

Tibia

Tibialis anterior

Extensor carpi ulnaris

Imprint / Impressum

Digital Front GmbH
Mergenthalerallee 73-75
65760 Eschborn
Deutschland (Germany)

E-Mail: info@digital-front.de

Representatives / Vertretungsberechtigte:
Alexander Mendelson, Leonid Ravin

Address / Anschrift:
Mergenthalerallee 73-75
65760 Eschborn
Deutschland (Germany)

Made in United States
Troutdale, OR
12/17/2023

15991534R00058